HERBAL ANTIBIOTICS

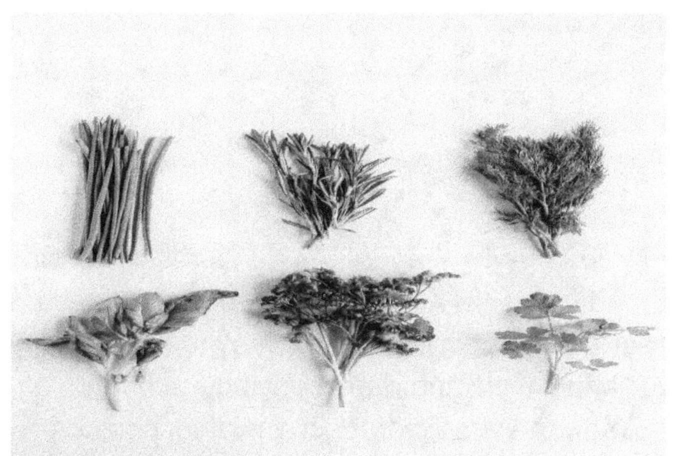

A complete guideline to Unlock natural medicine to prevent and cure drug- resistance bacteria and help boost your well-being

Avila Wanda

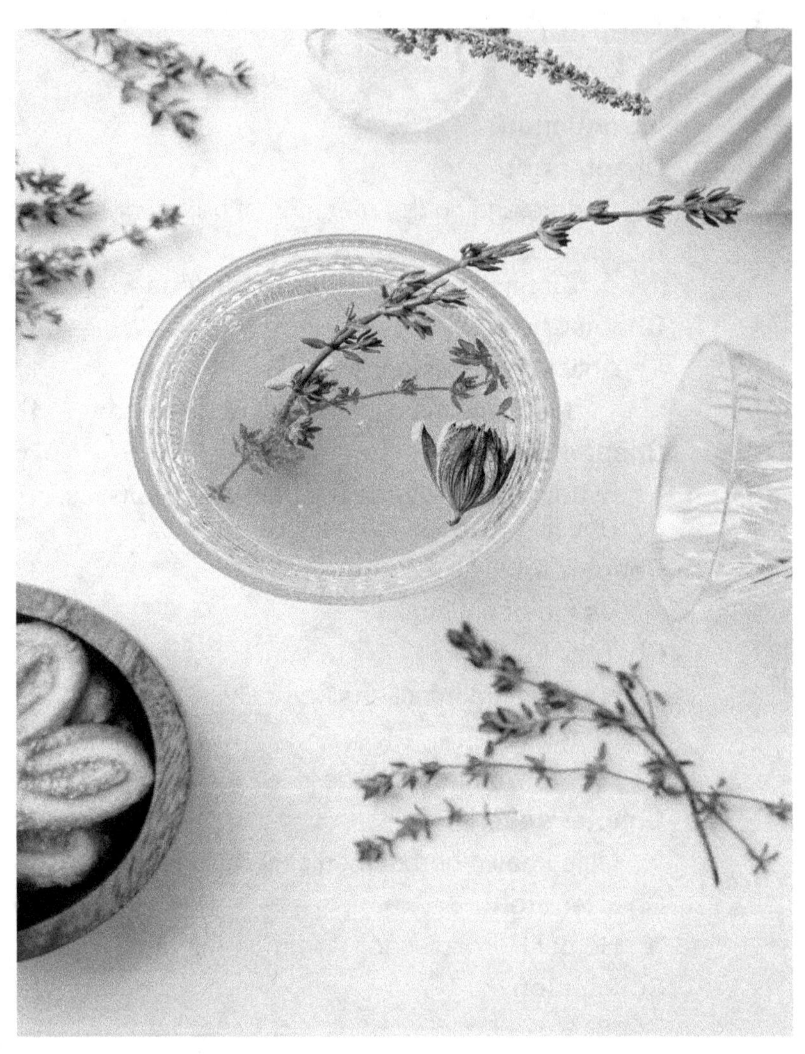

Introduction

In a world increasingly reliant on pharmaceutical solutions, a quiet revolution has been brewing in the form of herbal antibiotics. As the veil of modern medicine is lifted, ancient remedies rooted in nature are regaining their relevance. In the heart of this resurgence lies a tale of resilience and rediscovery.

Amidst the towering concrete structures and sterile laboratories, there exists a community that holds the secrets of herbal healing passed down through generations. In the quaint village of Verdura, nestled between emerald hills, an apothecary named Avila unveils the power of herbal antibiotics.

Avila, with her weathered hands and a twinkle in her eye, inherited the age-old wisdom of plant-based medicine from her grandmother. Her small shop, filled with jars of dried herbs and elixirs, becomes a haven for those seeking an alternative to synthetic antibiotics. In this tale, the herbs themselves become characters, each with its own story and ability to combat ailments.

The village faces a health crisis as a mysterious illness sweeps through, resistant to conventional antibiotics. Desperation leads the afflicted to Avila's doorstep, where she draws upon the medicinal properties of herbs like garlic, echinacea, and oregano. The villagers witness the miraculous recovery of their loved ones, and soon word spreads beyond Verdura.

Herbal antibiotics, once dismissed as folklore, gain recognition as a viable and potent solution. The narrative unfolds as more communities embrace the synergy between traditional wisdom and scientific validation. The story weaves through laboratories where researchers diligently study the mechanisms of herbal compounds, connecting the ancient practices with modern understanding.

In the realm of herbal antibiotics, a tapestry of knowledge, culture, and nature intertwines, offering humanity a path back to the healing embrace of the earth. The story of Verdura becomes a metaphor for a global shift, reminding us that within the roots and leaves, nature holds the keys to our well-being.

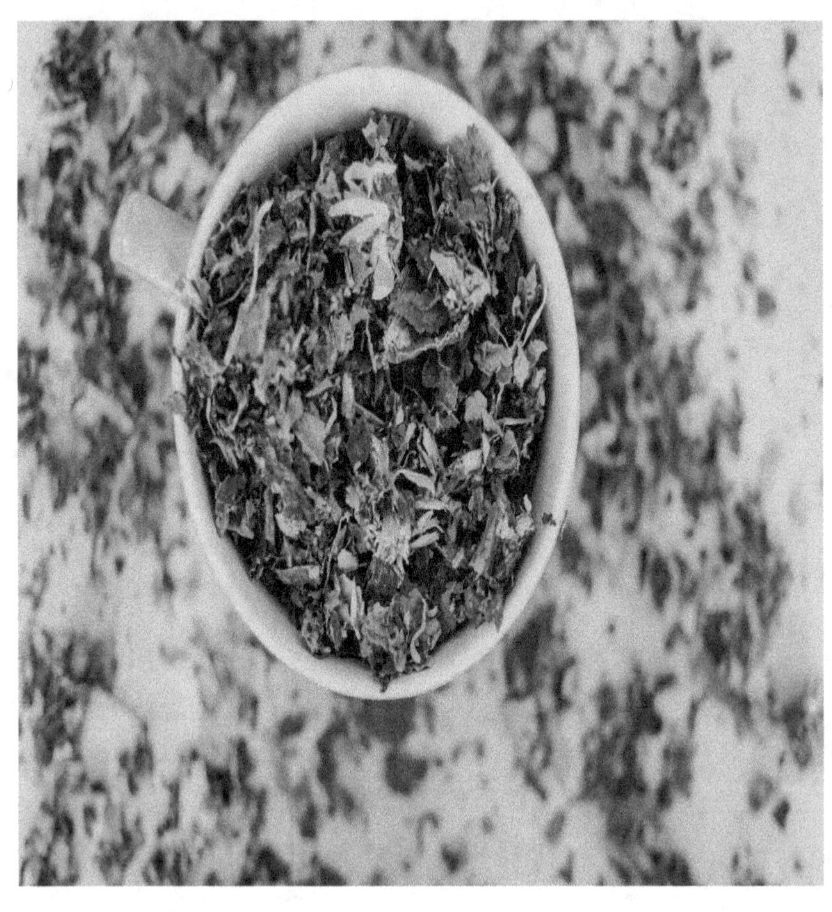

Chapter one

Understanding the meaning of herbal antibiotics

Herbal antibiotics refer to natural substances derived from plants that exhibit antimicrobial properties, capable of combating bacterial infections. Unlike conventional antibiotics synthesized through chemical processes, herbal antibiotics harness the healing power of various plant compounds to target and eliminate harmful bacteria.

These plant-based alternatives have been used for centuries in traditional medicine systems around the world. The term encompasses a wide range of herbs and plants known for their antimicrobial, antiviral, and antifungal properties. Examples include garlic, echinacea, oregano, thyme, and turmeric, among others.

Herbal antibiotics work through diverse mechanisms, such as disrupting bacterial cell walls, inhibiting protein synthesis, or interfering with essential metabolic processes within the bacteria. The complexity of plant compounds allows for a broader spectrum of action, potentially addressing a variety of bacterial strains.

In recent times, the resurgence of interest in herbal antibiotics is driven by concerns over antibiotic resistance and the desire for more sustainable and natural healthcare solutions. Research has delved into understanding the specific bioactive compounds in these herbs, shedding light on their potential as effective alternatives to synthetic antibiotics.

It's important to note that while herbal antibiotics can offer valuable therapeutic effects, they are not a panacea, and their use should be approached with caution. Consulting with healthcare professionals is crucial to ensure proper dosage, potential interactions, and suitability for specific health conditions. The exploration of herbal antibiotics represents a harmonious blend of traditional wisdom and modern scientific scrutiny, offering a promising avenue for holistic healthcare.

Controversial facts about bacteria

1. Bacterial Resistance to Antibiotics: One of the most significant controversies

surrounding bacteria is their ability to develop resistance to antibiotics. Overuse and misuse of antibiotics in medical, agricultural, and veterinary practices have accelerated this resistance, posing a serious threat to human health as it limits the effectiveness of crucial antibiotic treatments.

2. Bacteria in the Human Microbiome: While bacteria are often associated with illness, many play vital roles in maintaining human health. The human microbiome is a complex ecosystem of bacteria, viruses, and fungi that inhabit our bodies. The controversy lies in understanding the delicate balance between beneficial and harmful bacteria,

challenging traditional views that categorize all bacteria as pathogens.

3. Gut-Brain Connection: Emerging research suggests a connection between gut bacteria and mental health. The gut-brain axis implies that the composition of bacteria in the digestive system may influence mental well-being and cognitive functions. This concept challenges conventional thinking that mental health is solely a result of neurological factors.

4. Biological Warfare and Bioterrorism: Bacteria have been weaponized throughout history, and the potential for their use in biological warfare and bioterrorism raises ethical and security concerns. The controversy lies in the dual-use nature of microbiology

research, where advancements intended for beneficial purposes could also be exploited for harmful intentions.

5. Bacteria as Agents of Evolution: Bacteria play a crucial role in evolution through processes like horizontal gene transfer. This controversial concept challenges the traditional understanding of evolution based solely on genetic inheritance, as bacteria can transfer genes horizontally between different species, contributing to genetic diversity and adaptation.

6. Bacteria in Space: The potential for bacteria to survive and thrive in space raises questions about the possibility of microbial life existing beyond Earth. Controversies emerge regarding the search for extraterrestrial life and the

potential risks of contaminating other celestial bodies with Earth-originated bacteria during space exploration.

These controversial aspects highlight the complex and multifaceted nature of bacteria, showcasing their capacity for both positive and negative impacts on human health, ecosystems, and scientific understanding.

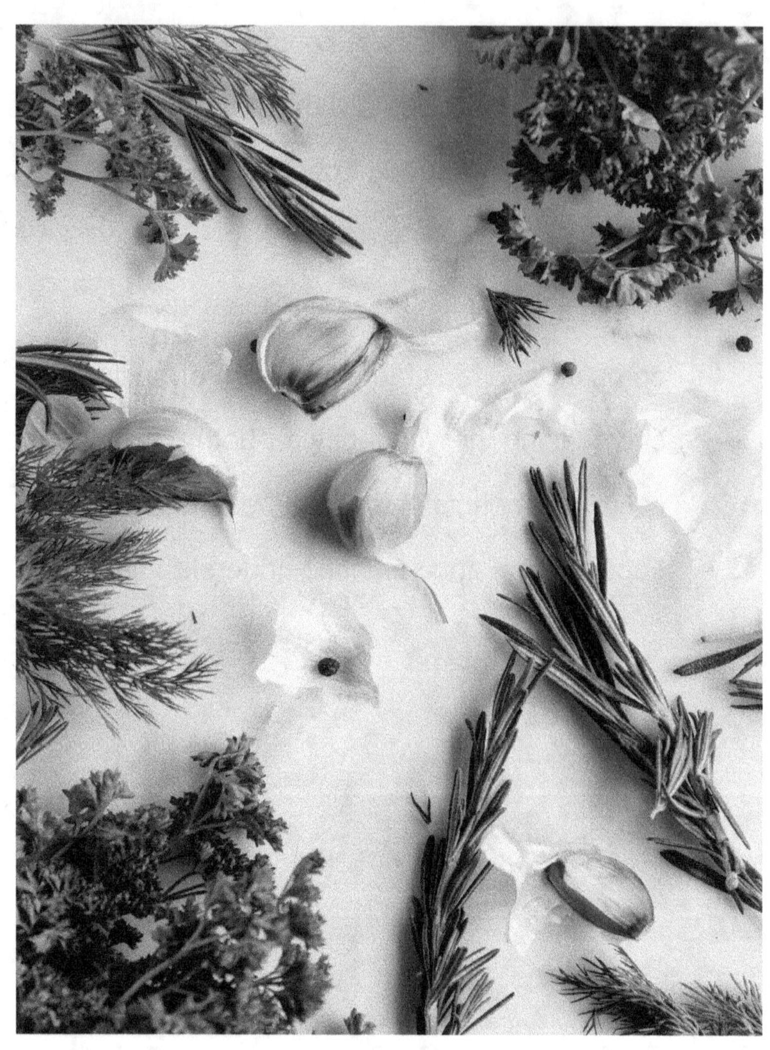

Chapter two

Antibiotics resistance

Antibiotic Resistance: A Growing Global Threat

Antibiotic resistance is a complex and pressing global health issue that arises when bacteria, fungi, or other microorganisms evolve to withstand the effects of medications designed to kill or inhibit them. This phenomenon has profound implications for human health, as it diminishes the effectiveness of antibiotics, rendering once-treatable infections more challenging to manage.

Mechanisms of Antibiotic Resistance:

1. Genetic Mutation: Bacteria can undergo spontaneous genetic mutations that confer resistance to antibiotics. These mutations may alter the target of the antibiotic or enhance the microorganism's ability to expel the drug.

2. Horizontal Gene Transfer: Bacteria can share genetic material horizontally, transferring resistance genes among themselves. This can occur through processes such as conjugation, transformation, or transduction, facilitating the rapid spread of resistance traits.

3. Overuse and Misuse: Antibiotic resistance is exacerbated by the

overuse and abuse of antibiotics. Incomplete treatment courses, unnecessary prescriptions, and the use of antibiotics in livestock feed amplify selective pressure, encouraging the survival of resistant strains.

Global Impact:

1. Increased Mortality and Morbidity: Resistant infections are associated with higher mortality rates and increased morbidity. Routine medical procedures, such as surgeries, chemotherapy, and organ transplants, become riskier when effective antibiotics are limited.
2. Prolonged Illness: Antibiotic resistance can lead to prolonged illnesses as conventional treatments become less

effective. Patients may experience extended hospital stays, increased healthcare costs, and a higher likelihood of complications.

3. Economic Burden: The economic impact of antibiotic resistance is substantial, affecting healthcare systems, productivity, and agriculture. Treating resistant infections often requires more expensive and resource-intensive interventions.

Drivers of Antibiotic Resistance:

1. Overprescribing: Inappropriate prescribing of antibiotics for viral infections or mild illnesses contributes to resistance. Healthcare practitioners, pressured by patient expectations or

diagnostic uncertainty, may prescribe antibiotics unnecessarily.

2. Agricultural Practices: The use of antibiotics in agriculture for growth promotion and disease prevention in livestock contributes to the spread of resistant bacteria. Resistant strains can be transmitted to humans through the food chain or environmental contamination.

3. Globalization and Travel: The ease of international travel and trade facilitates the spread of resistant bacteria across borders. Resistant strains that emerge in one region can quickly become global health threats.

Addressing Antibiotic Resistance:

1. Stewardship Programs: Implementing
    antibiotic stewardship programs in
    healthcare settings to promote
    responsible use, proper dosing, and
    duration of antibiotic treatment.

2. Research and Development: Investing
    in research to develop new antibiotics
    and alternative treatments to combat
    resistant strains.

3. Global Cooperation: Fostering
    international collaboration to monitor
    and address antibiotic resistance on a
    global scale, recognizing that the issue
    transcends national borders.

4. Public Awareness: Educating healthcare
    providers, patients, and the public about
    the responsible use of antibiotics, the
    consequences of resistance, and the

importance of completing prescribed courses.

5. Regulatory Measures: Implementing and enforcing regulations to control the use of antibiotics in agriculture and veterinary medicine, limiting unnecessary exposure and promoting responsible practices.

Addressing antibiotic resistance requires a multifaceted and coordinated effort at local, national, and global levels. The stakes are high, and concerted action is essential to preserve the effectiveness of antibiotics for current and future generations.

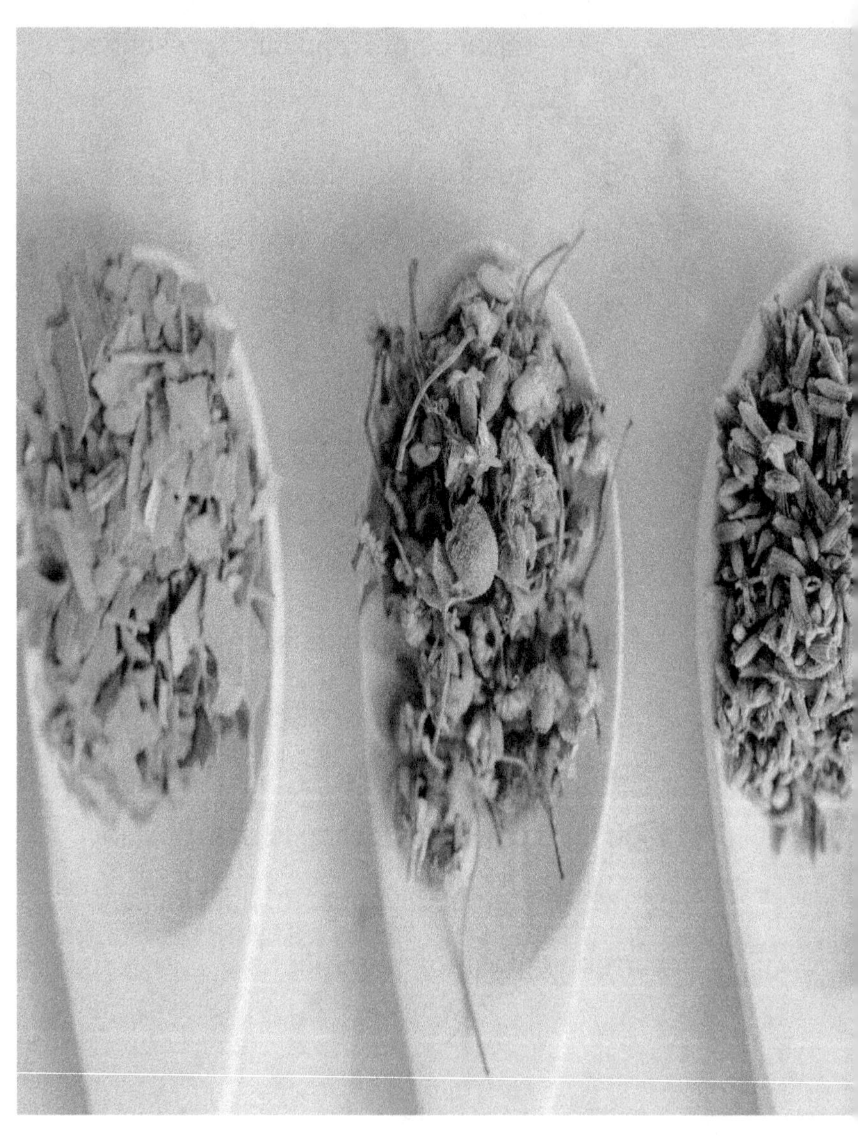

Chapter three

Eye-Opening Alternative Medicine Statistics: Unveiling Trends in Healthcare

1. Growing Popularity:

   - According to a National Health Interview Survey, approximately 33.2% of adults in the United States used some form of complementary or alternative medicine in 2017.

2. Global Acceptance:

   - The World Health Organization (WHO) reports that traditional medicine, including herbal remedies, acupuncture, and traditional healing practices, is widely used globally, with up to 80% of some populations relying on these approaches for primary healthcare.

3. Increased Spending:
   - A survey conducted by the National Center for Complementary and Integrative Health (NCCIH) revealed that Americans spent approximately $30.2 billion on complementary health approaches in 2012, encompassing practitioner visits, dietary supplements, and natural products.

4. Integration into Mainstream Healthcare:
   - The integration of alternative medicine into conventional healthcare is evident. In the

United States, more than 60% of medical schools offer elective courses on alternative therapies, reflecting a growing acknowledgment within the medical community.

5. Rising Use Among Cancer Patients:
    - Cancer patients are increasingly turning to alternative therapies. A study in the Journal of Clinical Oncology found that 40% of cancer patients use complementary and alternative medicine, often alongside conventional treatments, to manage symptoms and improve quality of life.

6. Mind-Body Practices on the Rise:

- Mind-body practices, such as yoga and meditation, have gained significant traction. The National Health Interview Survey reported that over 14% of adults practiced yoga in the United States in 2017, and meditation use nearly tripled from 4.1% in 2012 to 14.2% in 2017.

7. Herbal Supplement Use:

    - Herbal supplements are widely consumed. The Nutritional Business Journal estimates that sales of herbal dietary supplements in the United States reached $9.6 billion in 2019, reflecting a consistent upward trend.

8. Prevalence of Acupuncture:

- Acupuncture, an ancient Chinese practice, has seen increased acceptance. The National Health Interview Survey states that over 14 million U.S. adults had used acupuncture by 2017, marking a substantial rise in adoption.

9. Positive Patient Experiences:

     - Patient satisfaction with alternative medicine is notable. A study published in the Journal of General Internal Medicine found that patients who use complementary and alternative medicine often report improved health outcomes, with high levels of satisfaction regarding their healthcare experiences.

10. Global Perspectives:

- The use of traditional and alternative medicine is not limited to Western societies. In many Asian, African, and Latin American countries, traditional healing practices remain deeply embedded in cultural and healthcare systems.

These alternative medicine statistics highlight a shifting paradigm in healthcare, where individuals are increasingly embracing diverse approaches to promote well-being and address health concerns. As the popularity and integration of alternative medicine continue to grow, it prompts a reevaluation of healthcare practices and encourages a more holistic perspective on healing.

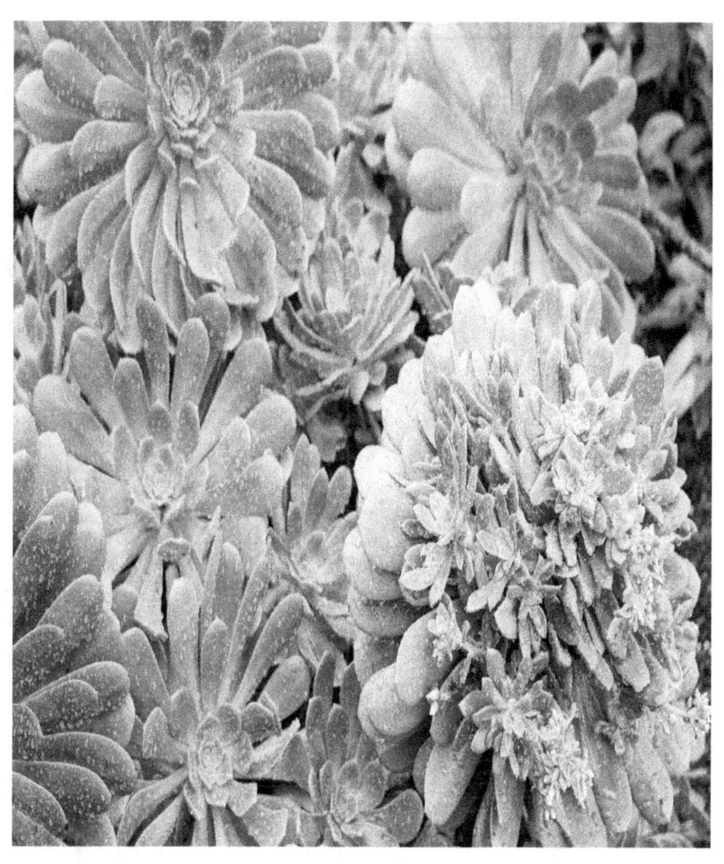

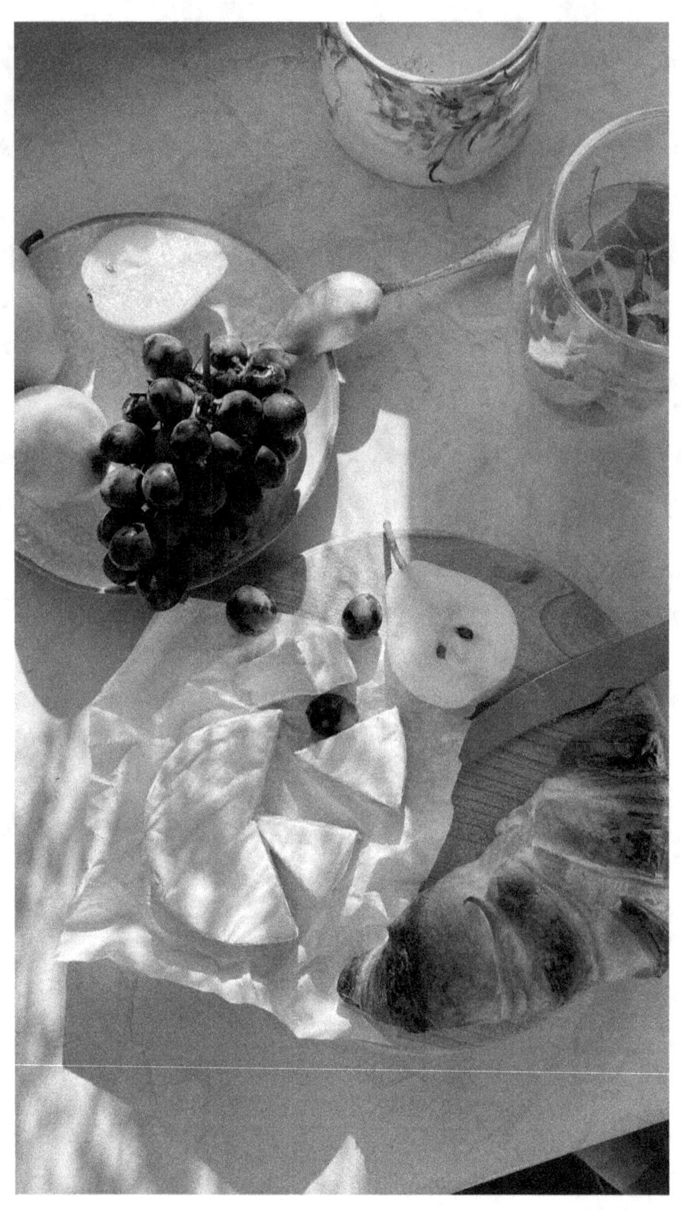

Chapter four

Usage of antibiotics

Antibiotics: All You Need to Know About Their Usage

1. What Are Antibiotics?

- Antibiotics are powerful medications designed to fight bacterial infections. They work by either killing bacteria or preventing their growth and reproduction.

2. Types of Antibiotics:

- Antibiotics come in various classes, each targeting specific types of bacteria.

Common classes include penicillins, cephalosporins, macrolides, tetracyclines, and fluoroquinolones.

3. When Are Antibiotics Necessary?

- Antibiotics are effective against bacterial infections but are ineffective against viral infections, such as the common cold or flu. They are prescribed by healthcare professionals when a bacterial infection is diagnosed.

4. Overuse and Misuse:

- Antibiotic resistance is a result of both improper and excessive usage of antibiotics. Completing the full

prescribed course is crucial, as stopping
early may leave surviving bacteria more
resistant.

5. Antibiotic Resistance:

- Bacteria develop antibiotic resistance
  when they adapt to resist the effects of
  antibiotics. It is a global health threat,
  making once-treatable infections more
  difficult to manage.

6. Common Infections Treated with Antibiotics:

- Antibiotics are commonly prescribed for
  respiratory infections (such as
  pneumonia and bronchitis), urinary tract
  infections, skin infections, ear infections,

and certain sexually transmitted
infections.

7. Side Effects:

- Antibiotics can have side effects, ranging from mild to severe. Allergic reactions, diarrhoea, and nausea are typical adverse effects.It's essential to inform healthcare providers of any allergies or adverse reactions to antibiotics.

8. Interactions with Other Medications:

- Some antibiotics may interact with other medications, affecting their effectiveness or causing adverse reactions. Tell medical professionals about all of your prescriptions, including over-the-counter medicines and dietary supplements.

9. Probiotics and Gut Health:

- Antibiotics can disrupt the balance of beneficial bacteria in the gut, leading to conditions like antibiotic-associated diarrhea. Probiotics may be recommended to restore gut health during and after antibiotic treatment.

10. Pregnancy and Antibiotics:

- While certain antibiotics are safe to use while pregnant, others may be dangerous. It's crucial for pregnant individuals to discuss antibiotic use with their healthcare provider to ensure the well-being of both mother and baby.

11. Completing the Prescribed Course:

- To prevent antibiotic resistance, it's essential to complete the full prescribed course, even if symptoms improve before the medication is finished. Early termination may make remaining germs more resilient.

12. Importance of Healthcare Professional Guidance:

-It is important to utilize antibiotics only under a doctor's supervision. Self-prescribing or sharing antibiotics is strongly discouraged, as it can lead to inappropriate use and contribute to resistance.

Understanding antibiotics, their appropriate use, and the potential risks and benefits is crucial for promoting both individual and public health. Responsible antibiotic use plays a vital role in mitigating antibiotic resistance and ensuring the continued effectiveness of these life-saving medications.

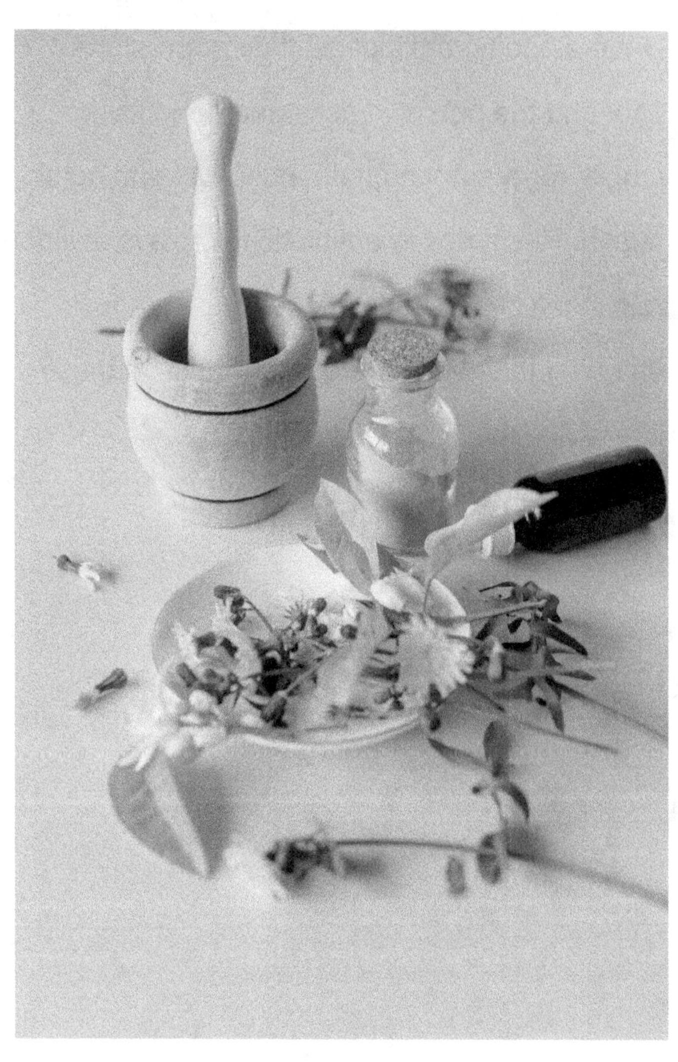

Chapter Five

How to fight infections naturally

Natural Approaches to Fight Infections:

Supporting Your Immune System

1. Healthy Diet:
   - Eat a diet high in fruits, vegetables, whole grains, lean proteins, and balance.Nutrients such as vitamin C, zinc, and antioxidants support the immune system.

2. Hydration:
   - Stay well-hydrated by drinking plenty of water. Adequate hydration helps flush toxins from

the body and supports overall health.

3. Adequate Sleep:

    ○ Ensure sufficient, quality sleep. An effective immune system depends on getting enough sleep. Aim for 7-9 hours of sleep per night.

4. Regular Exercise:

    ○ Engage in regular, moderate exercise. Physical activity promotes circulation and contributes to overall health, which can help the immune system function optimally.

5. Stress Management:

    ○ Engage in stress-reduction practices like yoga, deep breathing, and meditation.

Prolonged stress impairs immunity, increasing the body's susceptibility to illnesses.

6. Probiotics and Fermented Foods:

    o   Incorporate probiotics into your diet through foods like yogurt, kefir, and fermented vegetables. Probiotics support gut health, which plays a crucial role in overall immune function.

7. Herbal Remedies:

    o   Explore herbal remedies with known immune-boosting properties, such as echinacea, elderberry, garlic, and ginger. These herbs have been traditionally used to support the body's defense against infections.

8. Garlic:

- Garlic is renowned for its antimicrobial properties. Incorporate fresh garlic into your meals or consider taking garlic supplements (after consulting with a healthcare professional).

9. Vitamin D:

- Ensure adequate vitamin D levels. Sunlight exposure, fortified foods, and supplements can help maintain optimal vitamin D levels, which are essential for immune function.

10. Stay Clean:

- Maintain proper hygiene, which includes frequent hand washing, to stop the spread of illnesses. Proper hygiene is a fundamental

step in reducing the risk of getting
sick.

11. Essential Oils:

    ○ Certain essential oils, such as tea
    tree oil, eucalyptus, and oregano,
    have antimicrobial properties.
    Use them cautiously, such as in
    aromatherapy or diluted for
    topical application.

12. Stay Informed:

    ○ Stay informed about your health
    and potential exposure to
    infections. Knowledge empowers
    you to take proactive steps to
    prevent illness.

Important Note:

Always consult with a healthcare professional before making significant changes to your lifestyle or incorporating new supplements, especially if you have existing health conditions or are taking medications. Natural approaches can complement conventional medical care but should not be a substitute for professional advice and treatment.

Chapter Six

Top 45 wondrous herbs

1. Turmeric (Curcuma longa):
    - Known for its anti-inflammatory and antioxidant properties.
2. Ginger (Zingiber officinale):
    - A versatile herb with anti-nausea and anti-inflammatory effects.
3. Garlic (Allium sativum):
    - Renowned for its antimicrobial properties and potential cardiovascular benefits.
4. Cinnamon (Cinnamomum verum):
    - Beyond its delightful flavor, it may have anti-inflammatory and antioxidant effects.
5. Lavender (Lavandula angustifolia):

- Used for its calming properties and pleasant fragrance.

6. Chamomile (Matricaria chamomilla):
    - Known for its soothing and calming effects, often used in teas.

7. Peppermint (Mentha piperita):
    - Aids digestion and can provide relief for headaches and nausea.

8. Echinacea (Echinacea purpurea):
    - Often used to support the immune system and reduce the severity of cold symptoms.

9. Rosemary (Rosmarinus officinalis):
    - Contains antioxidants and has been linked to improved cognitive function.

10. Sage (Salvia officinalis):

- Known for its antimicrobial
  properties and potential cognitive
  benefits.

11. Thyme (Thymus vulgaris):

   - Contains compounds with
     antimicrobial properties and is
     used in culinary and medicinal
     applications.

12. Oregano (Origanum vulgare):

   - High in antioxidants and
     well-known for having
     antibacterial qualities.

13. Basil (Ocimum basilicum):

   - Offers anti-inflammatory and
     antioxidant benefits.

14. Mint (Mentha spp.):

   - Refreshing herb with digestive
     benefits and soothing properties.

15. Ashwagandha (Withania somnifera):

- Adaptogenic herb known for its stress-relieving properties.

16. Holy Basil (Ocimum sanctum):

    - Adaptogenic herb with potential stress-relieving benefits.

17. Licorice (Glycyrrhiza glabra):

    - Used for its sweet flavor and potential anti-inflammatory properties.

18. Dandelion (Taraxacum officinale):

    - Known for its diuretic properties and nutritional content.

19. Nettle (Urtica dioica):

    - Rich in vitamins and minerals, often used for its potential anti-inflammatory effects.

20. Milk Thistle (Silybum marianum):

    - Traditionally used for liver health and detoxification.

21. Ginseng (Panax ginseng):

    - Adaptogenic herb with potential energy-boosting and stress-relieving properties.

22. Valerian (Valeriana officinalis):

    - Known for its calming effects and often used to promote sleep.

23. Astragalus (Astragalus membranaceus):

    - Used in traditional Chinese medicine for immune support.

24. Catnip (Nepeta cataria):

    - Known for its calming effects on humans and attraction to cats.

25. Fennel (Foeniculum vulgare):

    - Used for its digestive benefits and licorice-like flavor.

26. Coriander (Coriandrum sativum):

    - Adds flavor to dishes and may have digestive benefits.

27. Black Cohosh (Actaea racemosa):

   o   Used traditionally for women's
       health, particularly during
       menopause.

28. St. John's Wort (Hypericum perforatum):

   o   Believed to have mood-lifting
       properties, used in traditional
       herbal medicine.

29. Arnica (Arnica montana):

   o   Applied topically for its potential
       anti-inflammatory effects.

30. Cayenne Pepper (Capsicum annuum):

   o   Contains capsaicin and is known
       for its potential pain-relieving
       effects.

31. Yarrow (Achillea millefolium):

   o   used for its possible
       anti-inflammatory and
       wound-healing qualities.

32. Gotu Kola (Centella asiatica):

    o Used traditionally for cognitive
       support and wound healing.

33. Frankincense (Boswellia serrata):

    o Resin with potential
       anti-inflammatory and
       mood-balancing properties.

34. Myrrh (Commiphora myrrha):

    o Resin with potential antimicrobial
       and anti-inflammatory properties.

35. Hawthorn (Crataegus spp.):

    o Is high in antioxidants and
       promotes heart health.

36. Passionflower (Passiflora incarnata):

    o Traditionally used for its calming
       effects and as a sleep aid.

37. Skullcap (Scutellaria lateriflora):

    o Known for its potential calming
       and stress-relieving properties.

38. Mullein (Verbascum thapsus):

  o Used for respiratory health and
     soothing properties.

39. Red Clover (Trifolium pratense):

  o Rich in nutrients and traditionally
     used for various health benefits.

40. Ginkgo Biloba (Ginkgo biloba):

  o Believed to support cognitive
     function and circulation.

41. Burdock (Arctium lappa):

  o Root used for its potential
     detoxifying and skin-clearing
     properties.

42. Goldenrod (Solidago spp.):

  o Used for its potential
     anti-inflammatory and diuretic
     effects.

43. Moringa (Moringa oleifera):

- o Nutrient-dense herb with potential anti-inflammatory properties.

44. Saw Palmetto (Serenoa repens):

    - o Used for prostate health and potential hormonal balance.

45. Elderflower (Sambucus nigra):

    - o Traditionally used for respiratory health and immune support.

These wondrous herbs showcase the diverse world of botanicals, each with its unique properties and potential health benefits. Always consult with a healthcare professional before incorporating herbs into your routine, especially if you have pre-existing health conditions or are taking medications.

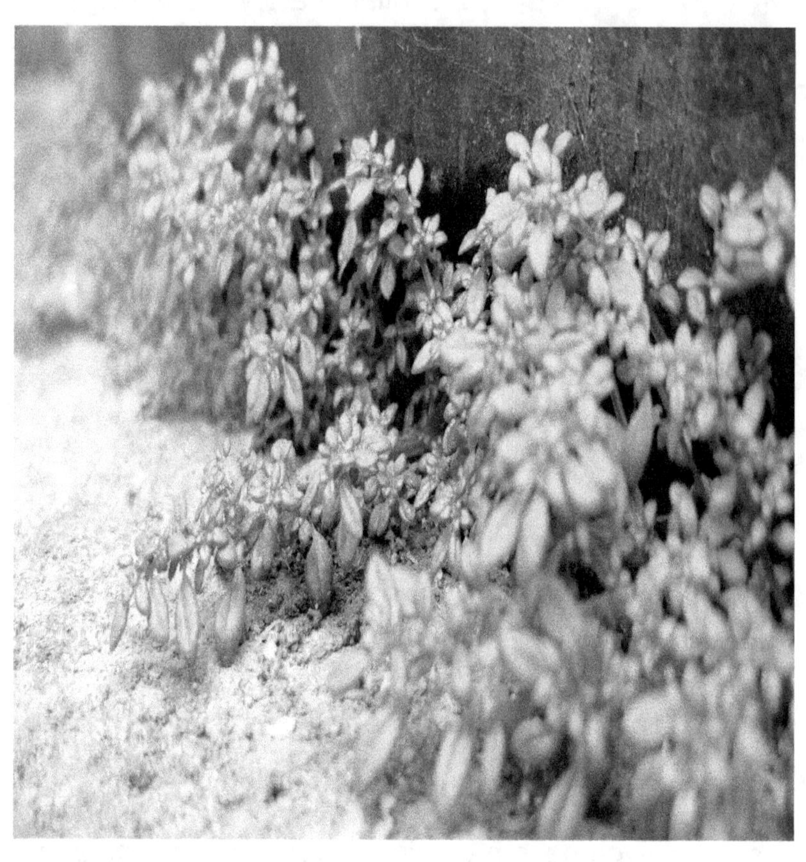

Chapter seven

Little known herbal medicine recipes

**1. Turmeric Golden Milk Latte:

- Combine 1 cup of warm coconut milk, 1 teaspoon of turmeric powder, a pinch of black pepper, and a touch of honey. This soothing beverage is known for its anti-inflammatory properties.

**2. Thyme Cough Syrup:

- Steep a handful of fresh thyme in hot water. Add honey and a squeeze of lemon. This homemade cough syrup

can help soothe sore throats and
suppress coughs.

**3. Calendula Healing Salve:

- Infuse calendula flowers in olive oil for a few weeks. Strain and mix the infused oil with melted beeswax to create a healing salve. Calendula is well recognized for its ability to soothe skin.

**4. Rosemary Infused Hair Rinse:

- Steep fresh rosemary in hot water and let it cool. After shampooing, use the rosemary infusion as a hair rinse. It's believed to promote scalp health and shine.

**5. Nettle Leaf Allergy Tea:

- Steep dried nettle leaves in hot water.
  This herbal tea may help alleviate
  allergy symptoms due to its
  anti-inflammatory properties.

**6. Chamomile Lavender Sleep Sachet:

- Combine dried chamomile flowers and
  lavender buds in a small sachet. Place it
  near your pillow to promote relaxation
  and improve sleep.

**7. Garlic Honey Immune Boost:

- Crush a few garlic cloves and mix them
  with raw honey.Give it a day or two to

sit. Take a teaspoon daily as a natural immune booster during cold and flu seasons.

**8. Minty Fresh Breath Tincture:

- Create a tincture by soaking fresh mint leaves in high-proof alcohol for a few weeks. Use a few drops as a mouthwash for fresh breath.

**9. Elderberry Gummies:

- Make elderberry syrup by simmering dried elderberries, water, and honey. Pour the cooled syrup into gummy molds for a tasty immune-boosting treat.

**10. Burdock Detox Tea:

- Steep dried burdock root in hot water. This herbal tea is believed to have detoxifying properties and may support liver health.

**11. Cilantro Heavy Metal Detox Smoothie:

- Blend fresh cilantro, pineapple, and coconut water for a refreshing smoothie believed to aid in heavy metal detoxification.

**12. Juniper Berry Joint Salve:

- Infuse juniper berries in olive oil, then mix with melted beeswax. This salve may be massaged onto joints for potential relief from arthritis or muscle discomfort.

**13. Hibiscus Rose Anti-Anxiety Elixir:

- Combine dried hibiscus flowers and rose petals in hot water. Add a splash of honey for a calming elixir believed to reduce anxiety.

**14. Fennel Seed Digestive Bitters:

- Steep fennel seeds in high-proof alcohol. A few drops before meals may support digestion.

**15. Lemon Balm Cooling Lotion:

- Infuse lemon balm leaves in almond oil and mix with melted shea butter for a cooling lotion. Apply to the skin for potential relief from sunburn or skin irritation.

When creating and using herbal remedies, it's crucial to be aware of individual sensitivities and consult with a healthcare professional, especially if you have underlying health conditions or are taking medications. Herbs may not be right for everyone and can cause

drug interactions.

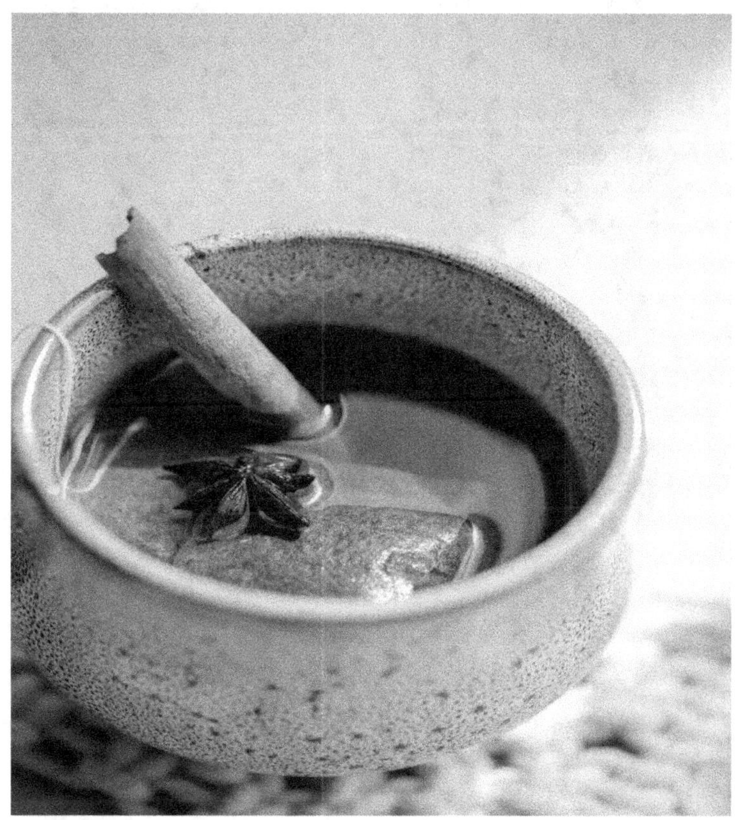

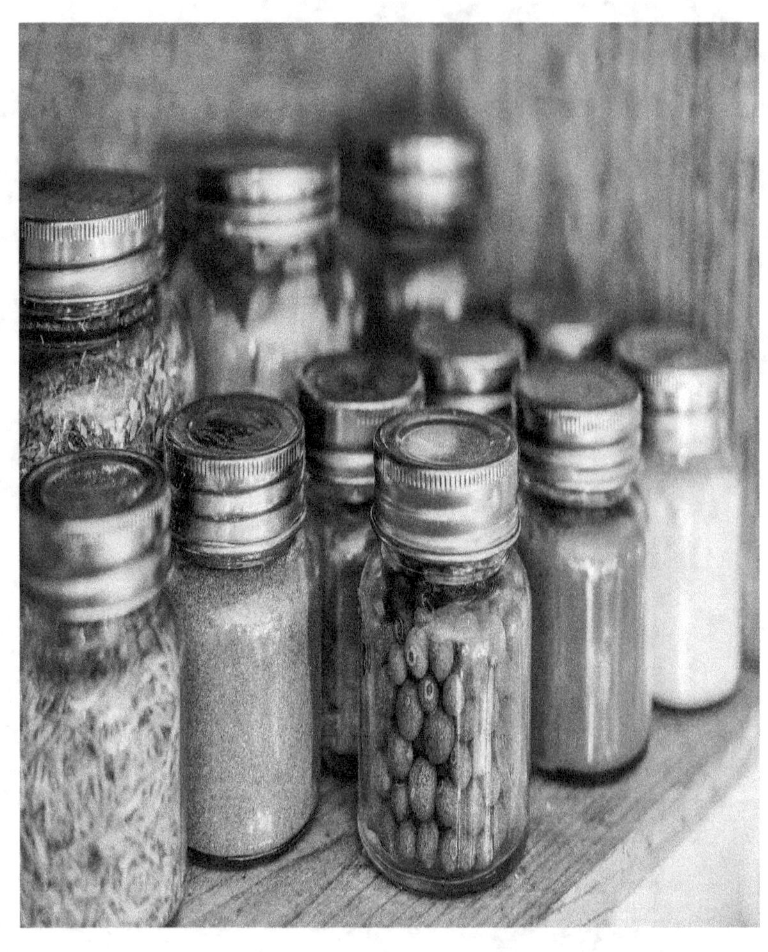

Chapter eight

Herbal Remedies for Common Ailments

**1. Cold and Flu: Echinacea Tea

- Echinacea is known for its immune-boosting properties. Steep echinacea tea with honey and lemon to help alleviate symptoms of the common cold or flu.

**2. Headache: Peppermint Oil

- Apply diluted peppermint essential oil to the temples and massage gently. Peppermint oil is known for its soothing properties and may help relieve headaches.

**3. Indigestion: Ginger Tea

- Ginger has anti-nausea and digestive properties.Steep fresh ginger slices in boiling water to make a calming ginger tea. Sip slowly to ease indigestion.

**4. Insomnia: Chamomile Tea

- Chamomile has calming effects. Drink chamomile tea before bedtime to promote relaxation and improve sleep.

**5. Sore Throat: Honey and Lemon

- Mix warm water with honey and a squeeze of lemon. This classic remedy can help soothe a sore throat.

**6. Upset Stomach: Peppermint Tea

- Peppermint tea is known for its digestive benefits. Sip on peppermint tea to ease an upset stomach.

**7. Stress and Anxiety: Lavender Aromatherapy

- Inhale the scent of lavender essential oil or use it in a diffuser. Lavender is believed to have calming effects and may help reduce stress and anxiety.

**8. Cough: Thyme Honey Syrup

- Create a thyme-infused honey syrup by steeping fresh thyme in honey. Take a teaspoon as needed to ease coughs.

**9. Joint Pain: Turmeric Paste

- To make a paste, combine water and turmeric powder. Apply the paste to joints for potential relief from joint pain and inflammation.

**10. Nausea: Peppermint Aromatherapy

- Inhale the scent of peppermint essential oil or use it in a diffuser to help alleviate nausea.

**11. Allergies: Nettle Tea

- Nettle tea may help reduce allergy symptoms.
Steep dried nettle leaves in hot water and drink
regularly during allergy seasons.

**12. Minor Burns: Aloe Vera Gel

- Apply fresh aloe vera gel to minor burns for
its soothing and cooling properties.

**13. Muscle Pain: Arnica Oil

- Arnica oil, when applied topically, may help
relieve muscle pain and inflammation.

**14. Acne: Tea Tree Oil

- Dilute tea tree oil and apply it topically to
acne-prone areas. The antibacterial properties
of tea tree oil are well established.

**15. Bruises: Arnica Salve

- Apply arnica salve to bruises to potentially reduce swelling and discoloration.

While herbal remedies can be beneficial, it's important to remember that individual responses may vary, and consulting with a healthcare professional is advisable, especially if you have underlying health conditions or are taking medications.

Conclusion

In conclusion, the world of herbal medicine unfolds as a rich tapestry, offering a plethora of remedies for common ailments. From the immune-boosting properties of echinacea tea during cold and flu seasons to the calming effects of chamomile for a restful sleep, nature's pharmacy provides a diverse array of solutions. Incorporating these herbal remedies into our wellness routines aligns with the growing recognition of the importance of holistic approaches to healthcare.

The use of herbal antibiotics, such as the antimicrobial powers found in garlic, thyme, and oregano, represents a bridge between traditional wisdom and contemporary health needs. As we explore the potential of these natural alternatives, it becomes evident that the synergy between ancient practices and modern understanding can offer holistic and sustainable solutions to combat bacterial infections.

However, it is crucial to approach herbal remedies with a balanced perspective. While these alternatives showcase promising benefits, their efficacy may vary among individuals, and consultation with healthcare professionals is paramount. Moreover, understanding the context of herbal medicine within the broader landscape of health and wellness emphasizes the need for a comprehensive and integrated approach to our well-being.

As we embrace the wonders of herbs, let us trade with respect for the delicate balance between tradition and science. Through informed choices, we can tap into the healing potential of herbal antibiotics, recognizing their role in supporting a robust immune system and fostering a harmonious connection with the natural world.